Broken but Not Shattered

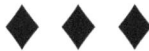

◆ ◆ ◆

I Found the Worth in Me

CHRISTINE NICHOLLS

ISBN: 9769547352
ISBN-13: 978-9769547353

Broken But Not Shattered

Copyright © 2016 by Christine Nicholls

First edition.

Unless otherwise identified, Scripture quotations are from the King James Version (KJV).

Published by CAB Publishing House

Kendal Hill, Christ Church, Barbados

Edited by RuthMoïsa Stoute of Moïsa Communications, Barbados and by Keisha Rodgers.

ISBN: 978-976-95473-5-3

CONTENTS

About this Book

Life is not about winning and losing. It's about winning and learning. I went through a difficult period in my life and to help me come to grips with my emotions I started to write. I found it therapeutic to say the least. As I assessed the various decisions I made during that dark period, I realized that others could perhaps benefit from some of the lessons I learned… and am still learning from my story.

'Broken But Not Shattered' takes you through my journey of looking for love, finding not quite what I had hoped for, and having to navigate life alone with anger, depression, and a brand new baby. Each chapter shares with you snapshots of what was going on in my life. Names of persons and certain details have been changed or left out, but generally, I do not hold back. I wanted to be real with myself… and with you, because this is the reality for so many women.

As you read, my hope is that I challenge you to be real with yourself, to examine your own emotional weaknesses and to ultimately find strength and purpose in the One who calls you worthy. God says in Psalms 139:11 that you are "fearfully and wonderfully made". He said that about you and me, knowing full well we were going to make a whole heap of mistakes in life. Our mistakes don't determine God's love for us.

You were created by Him to do something specific in your life, something He predetermined for you before you were born. You wouldn't go to a plumber if you were having electrical problems in your home. Neither would you go to a baker if you wanted to get your hair done!

We encounter so many unnecessary problems in life when we as women go searching in all the wrong places and all the wrong arms for our sense of identity and purpose. The person we should seek for those things is our Heavenly Father. I testify that because of His love and mercy in my brokenness, I have found the worth in me.

Introduction

Dreams

"Mummy, Mummy", my little girl screams, as she twirls around the room in her pink fairy dress and polka-dot leggings. Her "birthday girl" tiara perched on her head, she sweeps away the beaded braids covering her joyful eyes and dances in my direction. She grabs my hand and yells again, "Mummy, mummy".

"Yes, Janiyah! What is it?"

"Guess what I want to be when I grow up!"

"Hmm, let me see… a doctor, no, a teacher?" I ask, eyebrows now folded and one hand rubbing my chin.

"Nooooo, guess again, Mummy!" she giggles hysterically, tugging my hands in hers and pulling me around in a circle.

"A nurse… or a lawyer…?"

"Nooooo… Mummy", she now sings. "I want to be a PRINCESS! I want to be the prettiest princess in the world. I want to wear pretty dresses and live in a big castle. I want to *ride in a chariot with many horses. And everybody will love me!*"

***

Cinderella, Snow White, Sleeping Beauty, Ariel… fairy-tale princesses so many of us grew up reading about or watching on television. They were the prettiest in their lands. All eyes were on them. And even when they faced tremendous hardships – the tragic loss of loved ones or cruelty at the hands of the wicked – they somehow managed to overcome, or be rescued by a knight-in-shining-armor who would pledge his undying love and sweep them into happily-ever-after.

Fairy tales are for fools, some of you may say. But at some point in time, we all dreamt of what our happily-ever-after would be, could be. We wanted to be the prettiest, or smartest, or most loved, to grow up and be happy for the rest of lives…. Then one day, the wind of life blew with an unfamiliar rage, and some of us came tumbling down from the clouds to a hard, cold ground of frightful realities. Already bruised by the fall, uncaring feet kicked us around some more, until our inner resolve broke, until our desires turned into desperation, until we stopped dreaming of being princesses… or at least sharing those dreams, for fear of ridicule.

As a mother of two precious *princesses*, I'm eager to teach my daughters how to value themselves. I want them to know they were created to be loved and cherished, to respect others and to be respected. I don't want them to settle for less than they deserve. I don't want them to ever stop dreaming or believing that they are of great value, fearfully and wonderfully made by God who makes masterpieces.

Sadly, I lost sight of that fact in my own life… and more than once. I have had some knocks and bruises. My resolve to walk in my royal position was weakened. I feared. I stumbled. I nearly died trying to create my own version of happiness. Try hard as I might, I could not seem to arrive at happily-ever-after on my own. Like a princess who finds herself outside the protection of her father's kingdom, I eventually became bruised, battered and broken. I became an angry black woman imprisoned by misery and heartache. So empty. So lost. So unsure of my own value. I felt used and worthless.

I thank God every day that my story did not end there. No story has to end there, not yours… not the woman sitting next to you on the bus, nor the one at the school gate waiting for her children… not the woman who lives in the gated community, cut off from her family in the village nor the woman who earns so little she can't afford to leave the village. None of their stories has to end in despair and defeat. I thank God for being that light and comfort on the coldest of nights, and in the roughest storm. My flaws were before Him (still are), my hurts exposed and all my disappointments hung around me. And He still loved me. He helped me to find the worth in me. He helped me to dream again.

Chapter One

Red Flags

I once read a quote by Ebrahim Aseem[1], a writer and mentor for young black men in the United States. He said, *"Women will see red flags and stay years waiting for a man to reach potential."*

I think this is a remarkable trait for women to have... that is, the part about sticking it out for years in order to see someone else reach their potential. Now before you strike me off as being crazy, hear me out. There is something inside of every woman, something that sees what cannot be seen and hopes for the impossible, something that's willing to overlook flaws in order to reach the treasure in others. Women were created to nurture dreams and build societies. We do this for our men. We do this for our children. And we should be doing this for ourselves.

Knowing how to manage red flags (including knowing when managing is no longer an option and you need to walk away) is far different from pretending they don't exist. Red flags are actions, words, or events that point to character flaws in others and also in ourselves. We can't afford to ignore them because they point to an underlying and more serious problem. Sometimes we pretend for so long that we actually believe they don't exist. In this false sense of reality, how can we expect to make good choices or judge accurately when it comes to someone's character... including our own? It's quite simple. We don't!

Refusing to deal with red flags will not make the problem go away. What it does is keeps us in a state of disillusionment, believing that all is well. This is what I found myself doing, ignoring red flags yet again because I feared being alone. That fear branched off into several emotional weaknesses that caused me to make bad choices as I tried to "hold it down" and keep my man happy.

***

I was first introduced to Paul by a mutual friend. Eighteen years my senior, he would fit in with that subconscious ideal I had in my mind, of a mature man who could rescue me from a past of failed relationships and give me what I wanted; love and a happily-ever-after family. A single mom with a bruised heart, I had every right to be hesitant. Eventually though, with prompts from my friend to stop moping around, I decided there was enough there to give a relationship with this man a try. I wouldn't call it "love at first sight", but sparks began to fly almost immediately.

Our first date was at a popular restaurant on the not-too-busy south coast of the island. I paid great attention to how I looked that evening. Flowing curls framed my immaculately made-up face, my short stature boosted several inches by heels and a slimming outfit that hugged my curves in all the right places, revealing only enough to ensure Paul's eyes were on me for the entire dinner. Yet if anyone was mesmerized, it was probably me. Was it the magic of his expensive cologne which made me weak in the knees? Was it the stunning view of the sea from our table on the balcony? Was it the soft, sensual music of a live band playing in the background? Whatever it was, I was like Alice going down the rabbit hole. We talked for hours and hours, so eager to soak up everything there was to know about each other. That night was the most special I'd had in a long time. We were off to a fresh start and I was happy. Was I falling in love again?

Looking back, I'd say I fell pretty fast because in less than three months, Paul became a huge part of my life and I became part of his. After our first date we continued to meet, opening our lives to each other. Paul owned his own business and depended on me to handle some of its administration. I gladly did this. He made me feel like my opinions mattered. I couldn't hold back anything from him. I didn't want to. We talked. We shared. We had great sex. We held each other in our arms. I was in love and life was great.

Life was great, or perhaps I just really

wanted it to be. Things were certainly moving fast in the relationship, and too fast for my Christian upbringing. I had ideals, ideals of marriage, of connecting spiritually with a man who loves God and could help me live right. But needs were arising in me, stronger needs, and though marriage never seemed to be on the table for Paul, he seemed genuine and I felt I could let my guard down around him. He was present and I could depend on him financially and emotionally. He showed interest in my daughter and he could cook! I intended to make this one work for me.

So when time passed, and the first signs of trouble began to pop up, it wasn't that hard to ignore them and push aside that tingling feeling that my happy life was about to unravel. Paul's attention to me started to wane. He still showered me with gifts and knew when to say and do the right things to turn my frown into a smile. And whenever I thought he was misbehaving, I used my body to remind him of what he had… and my body was his weakness. But I would learn yet again that when it came to men, a woman's physical charm is not enough to keep him happy.

Paul's birthday was around the corner and I eagerly looked forward to celebrating it with him. I conjured up exciting plans and thoughts on how I should make that day an unforgettable experience. Extravagant dinner or a steamy getaway for just the two of us? Or should I buy him a gift. Shoes? Clothes? Cologne? Or a watch? I eventually settled on a pair of Kenneth Cole Jeans shoes and a matching shirt. I packaged them neatly in a gift bag with a birthday card. When I got home I decided to give Paul a call to talk about plans for that night.

"I don't feel like doing anything tonight," was his cold, dry response over the telephone. It was the furthest thing from what I expected but I

decided to keep cool and drop by his home later to surprise him with his gift. Maybe seeing me would change his mood. I noticed his moods were increasingly shifty. Maybe he was just stressed out at work. Maybe it was nothing.

Later that evening I arrived at Paul's home. The same Paul who told me he did not feel like doing anything for his birthday, was dressed up and about to leave. I walked over to him, a fake smile plastered on my face and presented him with his gift. He took it. No '*thank you*'. No peeking into the bag. Nothing. He shifted his attention to the television and began watching something. I turned and left. I was hurt and in tears but he was not going to see any of them.

A call from Paul several hours later moved me out of my coiled up, depressed state in bed, teary-eyed and disappointed. I was disappointed not only in how wrong the day seemed to be going, but because the wrong days seemed to be increasing. The heart-wrenching pain I felt from his don't-care-attitude and actions towards me was starting to glare me in my face. My stomach was in knots as I felt the boat of our relationship begin to tip. It seemed only I was trying to keep us afloat. I answered the phone.

Paul was on the other end and he spoke as if nothing had happened. No mention of the gift, nor of my earlier visit, nor of what happened between then and when he called. No apologies. I just listened to the sound of his voice as he went on about…. Slowly that sound caused my pain to go into remission. Thoughts of his arms around me flooded my mind. I couldn't think straight. What was the issue again? Each time I found myself in this position with Paul my inner voice would say, '*Why don't you call it quits before it's too late,*' but my fears of being left alone would reply, '*No,*

You're probably just crazy, if you settle down everything will be fine.' I was head over heels in love all over again with my man.

***

Women, that uneasy feeling in your gut, those tingles you get when someone is telling you something is the gospel truth but you know it's not, that little voice in your head, in the back of your mind that says don't trust him, that cautions you about falling in love, that shouts don't walk down that aisle and urges you to call the relationship quits if you want to live to see another day, aren't just fleeting thoughts to be tucked away in your subconscious. No... my sisters, they are warning signals from God, the One who created you and placed purpose on the inside of you. He is saying to you that where you are, what you are doing or about to do, is threatening to abort your purpose. You don't need a psychic to tell you something is about to go down. You don't need to be hooked on horoscopes. God's voice is reliable and He wants you to know you can trust in Him.

We often ignore what we feel and sense on the inside because we perhaps fear being alone or fear that the next man to come along might be a whole lot worst! As the old people say, "*you know what you got, you don't know what you will get*". For all we know, no one else better is going to come along, so we choose to settle. Sometimes pride makes us ignore those signs. We don't want anyone in our business. We don't want people to think we don't have it all together, that our love nest is far from loving…so we ignore the red flags and follow our heart.

Ladies, watch out! The heart can be tricky! Jeremiah 17:9 says "*The heart is deceitful above all things, and desperately wicked: who can know it?"* Your heart craves love and it will follow that path, but you must guard it from false love and guide it to a love God permits. After all, every woman wants to be loved, wants to express love, and of course wants to be able to call someone her own. But at what cost?

Chapter Two

Honoring our Bodies

Our body is a temporary house for who we are, from the moment we are conceived in our mother's womb, until the day we die. The way we treat it, and allow it to be treated by others, will have a direct impact on the quality of life we live. The bible says "*I will praise thee; for I am fearfully and wonderfully made: marvellous are thy works; and that my soul knoweth right well. My substance was not hid from thee, when I was made in secret...*" Psalms 139:14-15. God wants us to see our body as something marvelous. From what can be seen on the outside, to the complex way in which all of our organs, muscles, bones and even cells, function in harmony as we go about our day-to-day activities. Our body is worth our respect.

Failing to respect our body and failing to demand that others do so can point to deeper personal and spiritual issues. When we base our emotions on these personal and spiritual misconceptions, instead of God's view of our body, we make bad decisions (I'll talk more about emotions in chapter 4). A substandard perception of our body image, a belief that our bodies are tools to manipulate others, rather than temples - or even that we are slaves rather than masters of our own bodily desires - all lead us to making decisions that eventually impact negatively on our bodies. The following our signs that you could be doing any of the above:

- *Eating disorders*
- *Excessive exercise*

- *Food addictions*
- *Excessive, unnecessary reconstructive surgery*
- *Negative self-talk*
- *Depression related to body image*
- *Poor hygiene with no desire to improve*
- *Fear of seeing yourself in the mirror*
- *Habitual casual sex*
- *Drug addictions*

This list is far from exhaustive and I won't go into detail in this book. Also, my aim is not to judge or condemn anyone to whom these may apply, but for you to ask yourself what views of yourself and your body are you basing your decisions and emotions on.

I myself based my decisions on wrong ideas I had about the purpose of my body. I learned early on in life that a woman's body was power, a power she could use to bring any man to his knees. Though this is *true*, it is not a *truth* I should live by. I couldn't quite figure out why, even with all the power I thought I had, I still couldn't force a man to be loyal to me.

***

My birthday was a few days away and Paul has already agreed to take me to dinner. On the evening of that dinner date, Paul called to tell me he had loaned out his vehicle and would need a ride from work. I was baffled that he would choose to do something like that on such a special evening but I didn't want us to be late for dinner so I raised no issue and I opted to collect him. Two minutes into our driving, Paul shocked me once again, "*I am too tired to go out tonight*," he said. My heart sank. All my energy and joy were immediately replaced with deep frustration. As adrenalin rushed through my veins one question engulfed my mind. '*Am I not worth it?*'

When we reached his home, I rushed towards him screaming how much I hated him, how much he didn't care. I was angry, and in tears because he clearly did not care or was cheating on me. I deserved more. But my shouting soon turned into moaning. One touch and my heart melted. His lips were on mine, his body complimented mine. He whispered "I love you" and my body sank.

I used to think I knew how to play his weaknesses. Now I knew he had found mine. He could afford to take me for granted because each time he came around again, I would make it easy for him...

On the eve of a trip Paul was taking, he asked me to make some adjustments to his cell phones to avoid excessive charges and to ensure he could still conduct business efficiently. He gave me passwords for the devices, which I found to be very strange, and added a statement, *"I trust you Christine, you can have my passwords"*. Was this a test? If it was, I failed.

As quickly as I could, I placed one phone on silent and took a quick look at his messages, pretending that the transfers I was to complete were taking longer than expected. I was greeted by a stream of messages, all from women. I was hungry to read.

First message: *"Hi hon, I left the door unlocked for you"*. Not a message from me.

Next message, *"I love you, and I miss you, can't you come over tonight?"*

Next message: *"I love how it felt..."*

What the hell! How do men find the time to even cheat when you are with them majority of the time? I decided not to say anything.

During Paul's trip he called me every day to check up on me, telling me how much he missed me and how he couldn't wait to be back. His sweet words, his calling everyday seemed to hypnotize me and I began to miss him just as much. Paul really had game. He had me wound up so tightly that by the time he returned I was over at his house making love once more. My hopes for a fairy-tale relationship were over, but I did not want to let go. I couldn't, by this stage I was so addicted to Paul. My body belonged to him. I could not control my heart. I could not control my sexual desires and I was paying the price for it.

***

Ladies, the best part about our body is that it's here to help us to feel, to enjoy every single moment of our life. With our bodies we create life. We can touched and be touched by our loved ones. We can run around with our children, or hold them in our arms. We adorn our bodies to signify how we feel about ourselves and we walk a feet taller when someone compliments us on how great we look. And then there is the thrill of making love with a man than respects and values you, not just your body, but who you are. Our bodies are marvellous creations. God took the time to knit us together, from our heads, shoulders and breasts, to our hips, thighs and behinds. He took the time to make that complex organ called a vagina too! So why would we want to go and throw ourselves around with people who cannot appreciate us or our bodies, who see us as just one person on a list of several to "tick off"? If someone does not show you the appreciation you deserve, they should not be permitted access to the temple of your body.

So how can you ensure that access is denied to such a person? You must set boundaries, preferably *before* your sexual desires are aroused. Decide ahead of time against going certain places. Decide what an acceptable hour is for you or him to get up and go home... before you start to get too cosy and in desperate need of extra body warmth. Know your own sexual boundaries... and his! For some, holding hands is all it takes to get us sexually aroused. And stop trying to think you "can handle it". There's a fine line between handling it and being pushed over to the point of no return. A lack of boundaries is like leaving the door to our home unlocked: anyone, including unwelcomed guests, can enter at their will. Some men will pounce on you the first chance they get. Other men, the more devious kind, will tease you out, they will take their time in pushing back the boundary lines so that your desire keeps building under the surface. Before you know it, *you* are the one begging them to have sex! Stay away from them both. The man who is willing to wait to protect your virtue, to keep you untouched until he has paid the honourable price to be your husband, is the man you can consider keeping around.

It's not always easy, particularly when you have crossed that bridge already... and some of us have a really strong sexual appetite. But we must exercise control and not allow our sexual desires to cause us to enslave our bodies. In moments when you are feeling weak (what I really mean to say is *horny as hell!*) find something you love to do to bring your body under subjection and occupy yourself, preferably something that requires activity. Go for a walk or to the gym. Go cook or bake something if you like being in the kitchen. Sometimes just calling up a friend who can hold you accountable is what is needed.

1 Corinthians 10:13 tells us *"No temptation has overtaken you except what is common to mankind. And God is faithful; he will not let you be tempted beyond what you can bear. But when you are tempted, he will also provide a way out so that you can endure it."*[2] Pray and ask God to show you that way out so that you can endure, rather than give in. And when you do endure, you don't have to worry about feeling rotten, used, easy or gullible. Instead you feel like you have taken back your own dignity and self-worth.

Lastly, to those who believe in using their bodies to secure a man, here is a reality check for you. Manipulation is an act of a desperate woman. If you are underhanded in your attempts to "catch" a man, be willing to pay a far heavier price to keep him. Regardless of what you do however, if the relationship was not meant to be, your cheap tricks (or expensive shenanigans) will not work. So, let us as women stop treating ourselves like yesterday's trash, and let's reach out for something better!

Chapter Three

The Right Kind of Commitment

What are soul ties? Soul ties are intimate bonds between persons, created through some form of relationship. We have other expressions for it; a heart string, a soul connection, chemistry. Soul ties are formed between a mother and her child, between close friends or relatives, between lovers. Soul ties can be good. God cherishes wholesome, healthy relationships. They are the bedrock of a fully-functioning family and society. However soul ties can also be ungodly. These are created when we go about forming relationships outside of how God intended relationships to be, such as through all forms of abuse between two people, through fornication and adultery, and also through sexually perverse acts like incest. Ungodly soul ties tear down rather than build up, withdraw without replenishing, abuse rather than protect, suppress you rather than cause you to blossom. Ultimately, ungodly soul ties hinder you from walking in your God-giving purpose. It is hard to walk in God's light when we are tied to darkness.

Through disobedience, I tied myself to someone else in a way that was not God's intent for me... through sex with someone who was not my husband. Though it felt good for a while, my actions brought sorrow and a whole lot of complications, not only to my life, but to others. Sexual intercourse is a precious, God-created act which he reserved for marriage between a man and a women willing to commit themselves wholly to each other. The Bible says in Genesis 2:24, "*and the two shall become one flesh*". Our spirit, emotions and every aspect of our being is united with that person. We become glued to that person. When that relationship fails, the pain is like trying to pull away a piece of paper that has been glued to a card or wood. Even if you manage to remove most, there is always the extra bit that remains. It is stubborn. It does not easily come off. This is like some of us today. We have glued ourselves to someone, or to several persons, through sexual intercourse not permitted by God. And because God does not permit it, we can't expect Him to bless it. The relationship ends and we try to move forward... but we are broken.

On top of that, we have baggage stuck to us that eventually hangs over us like haunting shadows. What does this negative baggage look like? How do we know we are being burdened by it? We struggle to move on, our minds are constantly on replay and we keep reliving the past with that person. Our hearts are closed to anyone else. A closed heart usually is surrounded by bitterness, anger, resentment, hatred, even murder (if not the act, the desire to kill that person). Sometimes we are so broken by past relationships that we feel no one could ever love us. We have trust issues, we feel like everyone else to come into our lives will hurt or reject us. (See Chapter 7 on uprooting bitterness).

The result of these feelings is that we struggle to meaningfully commit ourselves to someone else. An inability to commit is a red flag that too many of us women try to ignore, or if we do recognize it, we try to fix it the wrong way. The problem is not the inability of a man to commit. The problem is the junk in his heart or the excess baggage in his arms that has him broken. Being a good woman won't keep a broken man, being pretty might barely get you through the door but won't help you to keep a broken man… and not even a baby is enough to help you to keep a broken man.

＊

During one of our telephone conversations, Paul asked me something that made my jaw drop to the floor. It wasn't the question itself, but the fact that of all persons, he thought to ask *me*!

"How can one person sleep next to another knowing that they are in a relationship with someone else?" he asked. I paused, I was confused. Where did this question come from? I noticed that Paul sounded stressed, he had become distant over the last week and was experiencing loss of appetite. He had been out from work on sick-leave leading up to this particular conversation. I figured that he had contracted the flu and that this was now taking a toll on his body. Was this strange question Paul or the fever talking? I asked him, *"how do you mean?"*

The response he gave me shook my entire world.

Her name was Sabrina, the mother of his son. *"Sabrina sleeps at me sometimes, yet she's in a relationship... and I am frustrated"* he cried to me... his current girlfriend. He continued to moan about her actions, asking me what it was she could be telling her partner when she spent the night over by him. Did he really remember he was on the telephone with me? I don't even know who was more naive. Him or me? I paused before I answered. *"How can you be upset if she has another man and we are in a relationship? Explain to me how you think I feel that another woman is sleeping at you."*

Apparently the fever broke just then, and he tried profusely to clean up his verbal spill, telling me I had it all wrong and that they slept in different rooms when she came over. I abruptly ended the call... but sadly, not the relationship. Guess I really did have fool stamped on my forehead.

The following day, Paul continued to reach out to me but I was cold towards him. This continued for a few days. Then, one day, with some of his friends present, I gave Paul an ultimatum: *"You have until the end of the month to make your decision, consider yourself lucky as I am willing to walk away from us right now!"* Not too long after, he called me over to his home and I went. There was a bag of clothes at his door which he told me had belonged to Sabrina. Paul then got down on his knees. My heart leaped. He began to beg for forgiveness, promising me to be a better man and thanking me for always being there for him. That's all he got down on his knees for, promises. But I so much wanted Paul to love me that promises looked really good. Maybe this was a start of something new. Something I always dreamt of. Something I thought I would never have with anyone else. I wanted so much to believe him and make us work. He burned me so many times. How could I truly trust him again? But was I willing to give him up?

There were times where we did not argue, times where we would both enjoy quality time, like our treasured drives to the country side. Times where we enjoyed eating out and having our own little silly talks. It wasn't just physical between us. This man had my heart. I couldn't detach myself from him just like that. But what about his own heart? Could he truly give me all of his heart? Sabrina's clothes were out of his house. But what about her? Was she still lingering in his heart?

**

Breaking free from ungodly soul ties becomes a whole lot easier when we purposely pursue God's best for us. Ladies, the standard God wants for us when committing ourselves to a love partner is to do so within the structure of marriage. This is not "old-school". This is God's only way as outlined in the Bible, our manual for living lives that please Him. Too many times we like to harp on about not being able to find a man who can commit themselves to us. And yet, we struggle to commit ourselves to God's best, to God's Word, to God Himself. We stray, our eyes wander, we get dragged away by distractions, we are not "fully there"… Does this sound familiar?

Let us get commitment in our hearts right before we try to drag commitment from someone else. Let our relationships be between two whole people who are individually committed to God and are walking in His best. This is a relationship or soul tie that God takes pleasure in blessing. But such a relationship can't happen if either party is broken. A broken person has his or her arms filled with negative baggage. There is no room for you… even if he or she apologizes 100 times there is no room for you so don't settle. Listen, there is a best for you. If you were the landlord of a house with a rental value of $1,000, would you settle for $500 from the first person that came along, just because he or she "looks good" or "seems nice"? Would you still not hold out for the full price?

Then let us ask ourselves, why do we settle for relationship agreements which fall far below the value of what we have to offer? Don't fall for someone who is just willing to throw money and dinners your way, but hasn't the slightest clue how to treat you with respect. Hold out for someone who is willing to pay the full price. Hold out for a man that loves God and who will, out of that love for God, determine in his heart to love you the way you deserve to be loved.

Chapter 4

When Emotions Trap You

I like Joyce Meyers because she keeps it real. She wrote a devotion called "We can't rely on Emotions to lead us the right way[3]". She said, *"...we have to be very careful not to be led by emotions. We need to follow something much wiser and much more dependable—and that is the Word of God"*.

Emotional weakness is not when we are void of emotions or emotionally drained. It refers to when we give our emotions so much power over our decision making (over what makes sense, over that tingling voice in our head or that gut feeling) that we are rendered helpless and must go along with them. The outcome is even more disastrous when those emotions or hinged on fear, rejection and low self-worth. Many times situations keep repeating themselves in our lives and we are not clear why. Why do we keep falling in the same area? Why do we keep attracting the same negative drama? It's because we keep making decisions based on these emotions which are driven by fear, rejection and low self-worth. How we break the cycle is by breaking the hold these three yokes have on us. It's not easy to do this, if it were I doubt anyone would choose to live this way. Sometimes the yokes become gripped around our necks because of an event that happened way back in our childhood. Maybe we were told that we were ugly, worthless, or that no one would ever want us. Maybe we were rejected by a parent or a spouse and never could figure out why. All we know is that we find ourselves at various points in our lives, afraid and unsure of ourselves. We find ourselves settling for less than the best because we don't think we deserve the best. We make tremendous sacrifices for others because we fear losing them if we don't. We tolerate others' perception of our own value because we have never defined what this is for ourselves.

God helped me to see that my decisions to hold on to something and someone that couldn't see the value in me was wrong. But even more importantly, that I let it happen because I did not know my own worth. Where did not knowing my worth originate from? Fear. Fear of falling apart if something did not work, fear of rejection, fear of not being understood, fear of not satisfying my partner and fear of being alone. My fear produced a low self-esteem within me. I became someone I did not want to be in order to get the love and approval I craved.

***

I still loved Paul. But I began to believe less

and less that I could make the relationship work, if what we had could still even be called a relationship. Take out the few bright sparks of our time together, and we were left with arguments, little trust and make-up sex. I was angry at Paul and blamed him of course. But my own emotions were continuing to blindside me and the decisions that followed left me in an even greater bind.

I met Mark online and a casual friendship developed. He was not my type but he seemed to show genuine interest in me despite knowing of my relationship with Paul. It was a very hurtful season of my life and Mark was the listening ear that I needed. He also encouraged me and made me feel like I was worth someone's attention, even if that someone was not Paul. Still for me, Mark was nothing more than a friend.

One day, while I was still at work, Mark called to tell me he was standing outside my office and that he wanted me to come down and meet him. It was our first time meeting face to face and though I couldn't understand why at the time, I was feeling jittery. As I opened the office door, there he was, standing with flowers in his hands. He introduced himself and we started to laugh hysterically. I started to feel more at ease and we chatted for a few minutes before I had to return to work. That visit turned out to be the first of many surprise stops by the office and often, Mark did not come empty-handed. I accepted his gifts graciously and it felt good to engage a man without any drama involved. Our friendship continued to grow.

Unfortunately, it was not long before I dragged Mark into my own drama with Paul. I was fed up with Paul but he still had full access to me. One early morning in particular I showed up at his house unexpectedly. I walked straight inside and allowed my eyes to wander around the room, looking for anything suspicious. I soon spotted damning evidence, but before I could interrogate Paul, he had already undressed me and we were in the act of making love. There, right under his bed, I spotted four pairs of female sandals. I gulped. My mind disconnected from my body as I remained silent. In the corner of my eye I could now see a set of women's accessories. Did this stuff mean that Sabrina was back? *"She never left! Why don't you wake up?"* I could hear a voice in my head saying. And then it happened. I heard Paul whisper to me, "I will never leave you Christine". I snapped. All the anger inside of me erupted and I pushed him from off of me. *"You already left, you liar!"* I screamed at the top of my lungs as I jumped off the bed and dragged the shoes from under it, like a mad woman. My head was hot. I hurriedly put on my clothes and barely heard him mumbling excuses. As I proceeded to walk out of his room, he stood in my path, tears now welling up in his eyes. I said nothing as I stared directly into his eyes. *"This is it Christine, now or never. Time to call it quits."*

I began to date Mark and I made sure Paul found out. He was furious and I confess I was loving this twisted form of attention. Two months into our friendship, Mark turned up the heat. He wanted me to meet his family. I felt sad. I was falling for him but I was also playing him by giving in to Paul's requests to see me. *"Oh! What a tangled web we weave when first we practice to deceive!"*[4] I couldn't even recognize who I was anymore at times. One night, Mark called me saying he had something serious to say to me. I invited him over and shortly after he arrived at my home, he shocked me by proposing to me. A diamond two-band gold ring stood there in his hand. I could barely see, my eyes were filled with tears. I had to tell him the truth. *"I can't, you know I can't, truth is I love two people at the same time. I still have feelings for Paul"*, I cried. Yet Mark insisted that I take the ring and think about what I really wanted before making up my mind. He left. That night was long. Mark was supposed to be a temporary distraction in my mess with Paul. Yet I loved him more than Mark who was offering me what seemed like what I wanted all along. *"God what should I do? Please give me a sign!"* I got none, so I cried myself to sleep that night.

The old people would always tell you, *"love who love you"*. So three days later, I accepted Mark's proposal and I called Paul to tell him I was leaving him for good. I told him of our engagement and in what seemed like less than five minutes Paul was banging on my door. He barged into the house yelling and asking me if I was crazy. *"You think you can sleep with me one night and the next day talk about you engaged to someone else?"* He pinned me to the wall, threatened to chop off my hand if he saw me wearing the engagement ring, and then marched out of the house.

I continued to see Mark but kept the relationship on a low profile. We were not sexually involved but he became very "protective" of me and would get angry when he found out Paul was still trying to contact me. I believed then that he figured that the ring I now wore meant he owned me. His persistent questioning about my status with Paul made me grow a little weary. I didn't want the stress from Paul and certainly did not want this from Mark. I began to think that maybe he was not the right man for me either.

***

Women can fall into the trap of making important decisions in the heat of the moment, when their emotions are clearly unbalanced. Unbalanced emotions are hardly ever rational. In my emotional state I rationalized deceiving someone else who showed genuine interest in me, I rationalized that physical and verbal abuse at the hands of a man possibly meant he still cared for me, I made a decision to marry when I could not even find my heart. Despite godly counsel I leaned on my own fears of being alone and a grasped frantically at any semblance of love that was being thrown my way. In the end I left a wake of destruction around me and had to find my way back with emotional scars and a back broken down by negative baggage. The fact that I had been down this road several times before clearly meant the defect was an internal one.

Ladies, allowing faulty or defective
emotions to dictate how we live our lives will
eventually lead us responding in panic and anxiety,
trying to appease someone we should in fact be
kicking out of our lives, and sinking into dark
depressing thoughts. The impact can only ever be
negative on our health and remaining relationships.
Simply put, you are setting yourself up for
disappointment. Like a ship on troubled waters you
keep being tossed side to side, back to front,
collecting water that will eventually cause you to
sink. The good news is that there is an anchor for
your emotions. You need something to base you
emotions on... something sure and steady to cover
your thoughts and feelings... positive affirmations
that you can use to wash and renew your mind.
Such affirmations can be found in the Word of God.
Sometimes we can also draw inspiration from the
lives and testimonies of healthy role models,
persons who have risen above fear and conquered
their own challenges. (I've included a section of
positive affirmations at the back of this book which

I recommend you use as daily declarations). Ultimately these affirmations are to help you to readjust your self-perception so that it falls in line with the perception that God, your Creator, has of you. They are to help you discover or rediscover your identity and your worth.

Yes, you are worthy, you have value, you are precious and you deserve to be treated as such! God does not see you as trash, something to be kicked around, and someone to be bought or traded for money, someone to be shackled and beaten. You are not cheap. But if you see yourself this way, you will subconsciously attract to you people who will treat you as such. Sometimes women ask the question, *why can't I find any good man? Why do all the men I date turn out to be monsters?* Well ladies, these men have a problem but the bigger problem, the one you can fix, is the problem of attracting and being attracted to the wrong type of man. Some of us will settle for being someone's *other*, and then be heart-broken that we cannot be that someone's *only*. We will keep making excuses for their abuse, and then wonder why they don't have any respect for us. Some of us are such emotional push-overs that the more disrespected we are by the men in our lives, the more we are willing to roll out the red-carpet treatment, all for the sake of having someone in our lives. Such a man will kill you! It may not be a physical murder, but it may be an emotional murder, a murder of your dignity and self-worth. Get out now! Respect and love yourself enough to walk away from anyone that adds no growth or happiness to your life. Respect and love yourself to know that God *loves you and has a best for you*. Now that is something you can anchor your emotions to!

Chapter Five

Children are a Blessing

A woman may love her children, while struggling to love herself. Sad as that is, it baffles me more when a woman hates her children, yet claims to love herself. I see my children as an extension of me, a continuation of a bond which began in my womb. But I confess, there were moments when I thought that bringing them into the world was not the best thing... that it would only complicate an already complicated life. Those moments are made all the more worse when you don't have the support from the father of the child.

Sometimes women see their children as inconveniences. To be fair to them, the timing might have been inconvenient because of a career or education. Or they may struggle to make ends meet and see another child as bringing greater financial hardship. Sometimes the child can be an inconvenience for the father or new partner in the woman's life. A man may force you to have an abortion, saying that he cannot "handle" a child right now. He may even try to give you hope by saying, "a little later and we will have a family". Maybe you have children from a previous relationship, and the new man in your life thinks that they take up too much of your time. He may find ways to get in between you and your children, such as encouraging you to send them to live with a relative so that you could focus on the relationship more. For other women, the relationship has gone sour, but not before leaving a child or children behind. The father has moved on and in order to make him pay, the woman stops him from seeing his children or uses his love for the children to manipulate him into spending time with her. She is the queen and she will sacrifice her children like pawns in order to keep her "king" in check.

All of these situations can put us in a real bind, particularly if we are not sure of ourselves and allow people to make decisions for us that we should be making for ourselves. This is why it is so important for us to be emotionally strong. As discussed in the previous chapter, when we are emotionally weak, we have a greater tendency to make rash, illogical decisions that don't line up to God's best for us and create a mess around us.

***

My period was late. But irregular menstrual cycles were the norm for me so I thought nothing of it. I was however experiencing some muscle spasms in my neck and shoulders which I supposed came from working long hours at the office. One day, the spasms became so overbearing that I decided to go to the doctor. He gave me some pain relievers but a few nights later I found myself in greater discomfort. This time around, my tummy felt like it was being twisting and my back, as though someone was ripping it in two. I could not sleep. I could not sit up. I was in tears. My only comfort was the floor. I figured it was the side effects of the tablets the doctor had prescribed. A random thought came to me to cross pregnancy off the list of things that could be wrong, even though it was the farthest thing from my mind. Morning came and I stopped at a convenience store to buy the cheapest over-the-counter test. *It wouldn't hurt to just take it as I am sure I am not pregnant*. I took the test and placed it on the bathroom counter only to watch two strokes appear.....GULP!!.....no...this cannot be right. Was I really pregnant? It's probably just a false positive I assumed.

Yet that night I was worried. So many things flowed through my mind. How was I going to tell Mark, the man I was engaged to, that I was having

Paul's baby? How was I going to break the news to my parents and what would Paul's reaction be? I wanted morning to come so fast. I needed to find the truth. Was this baby a sign that I was to be with Paul? The following day I visited my pharmacist. I showed him the test. He confirmed I was definitely pregnant. My worst nightmare was happening. Still shocked, I said to him "*I will take another test*". He laughed at me and said, "*You can have a false negative but never a false positive*". I shook my head in disbelief and walked out with another test. I was hoping for a different result but the only change that time around was that the color of the lines was darker.

Paul and I were not on good speaking terms but I decided to break the news to him sooner rather than later. I showed him the test and his reaction shocked me more than the unexpected pregnancy. His first instinct...his first piece of advice...the only words I remember him telling me that day, "*Abort the baby.*" My heart sunk even further. Was this the man I really loved? I got up in tears and left his home without saying another word.   No amount of spasms I had felt up to this point compared to the pain I now felt. It emanated from my heart and caused shockwaves throughout my entire body. I could feel a dark cloud of misery hanging heavily over my shoulders.

The weeks to follow were hell. Paul called me again and again wanting more proof that I was really pregnant. He even purchased abortion pills for me to take and when I told him off, he decided to "punish" me by refusing to speak to me. When I eventually worked up the courage to tell Mark and to turn to him for some semblance of comfort, I found none. Instead, what I got from him was a recommendation of a doctor who performs abortion. *Abortions! Abortions! Abortions! Why do all the men in my life want me to kill my child?*

Believe it or not I still did what I could to cling to Paul, hoping that I could fix things. I had made up in my mind that this child was a sign that Paul and I were not history as yet and that there could be no future with Mark, me and another man's baby. Not wanting to have another child whose father was not actively involved in its life, I entertained thoughts of actually going ahead with an abortion. *Why is my fairy-tale not happening? I just want to be happy.* Sadness engulfed me to the point where I could not tell the difference between physical pain and emotional pain. At this point I was just into my second trimester and I began spotting. I was so scared. Was I losing my child? Did it decide to abort itself? I rushed to the hospital. My pressure was extremely out of control and as a result, I was given medication and had to report to the hospital on a weekly basis. Despite my mental and emotional state adversely affecting my health and that of my unborn child, I could not shake the depression, anger and bitterness growing in my heart. I rarely left the house, spent the majority of time in bed, ate infrequently and devoted quite a bit of my free time to crying. It was a pity party of one. I wanted to be alone in this world.

***

The key to being a better parent to our children in times of adversity, is to separate them from the circumstances. Being able to do this will call for emotional strength and a recognition that your child, just like you, was created by God. That child is fearfully and wonderfully made. That child should not have to pay for your sins or that of its father.

The Bible says in Psalms 127: 3 that *"children are a gift from God, they are a reward from him"*[5]. That applies to children who resemble the one who broke your heart, as was my case with this new baby. It takes courage and resilience to raise a child who was conceived in a season of pain. But I want you to know, God is merciful. He can give you joy in exchange for your sorrow. I know that in these seasons of pain, having an abortion can seem like the only way out. And I know that there is a great pro-choice lobbying effort to make us think that it is a viable option. But don't let us make decisions for the now, without thinking about the consequences to come later. If more women were honest, they would tell you that having an abortion may have made things easier for them, but it also left them to cradle another kind of unwanted baggage in their arms; resentment towards their partner, unforgiveness towards others and themselves for having taken a life, and shame. If this is where you are today, I want you to know that God is more than willing to lift you from this place of brokenness. You are still of worth to Him. He still sees value in you.

To those of you who may be, or know someone who may be considering aborting a child, please, I urge you, a baby is a miracle from God. Separate the value of that unborn child from your circumstance. Circumstances can change… and even if they don't change enough for you to ably mother a child, remember, there are other families who cannot have children of their own (or may just have the means to handle a growing family) and would be more than happy to raise this child.

Chapter Six

Don't Burn Your Bridges

Much of my story up to this point has been about me, Paul and Mark, about the swirl of confusion I found myself in and about how frustrated, lonely and unloved I felt. In that season of my life it felt like we were the only persons existing. Sometimes we get so caught up in our own bubbles of misery, we often exclude from that space, the people in our lives who truly love us and are always there for us. We find ourselves feeling alone when situations arise because all along the way to that point in our lives, we were subconsciously, or even intentionally, telling our loved ones to mind their own business and butt out of our affairs. They had their opinions, they meant well and shared their concerns from a place of wisdom, but we did not want to hear.

So we burned the wrong bridges and we built a fence around us. Don't get me wrong, fences are necessary to help us control what and who are able to exercise influence within the boundaries of our homes, relationships and lives. The worst thing you could do for your relationships is to let them be directed by everyone else's opinion. However, we must cherish and carefully consider the guidance of godly authority in our lives such as our parents, a relative or a teacher who has already shown a genuine interest in our lives, a devoted church leader and our close friends. What I've learned in my journey is that even though families can be crazy sometimes, they are God's gift to us. When the fire was out, and the smoke cleared, it was my family that stood by me to help me begin to pick up the pieces.

***

I made all the necessary preparations for the coming of my second child, in terms of the necessary material things. What I was completely unprepared for however was the fact that I would have to give birth to my baby alone and in extreme circumstances with mere hours determining if either or both of us would even live through the birth. I was barely 35 weeks pregnant. Nausea and pain had overtaken my body and I could not figure out if I was experiencing Braxton Hincks or real contractions. I took my blood pressure on a home device. It read 170+/150+. It was probably the pain I assumed... an indication that delivery was only weeks away. I'd been down this road before...no need to rush to the hospital I thought. As the pain intensified, I tried to wait it out, wishing it would go away soon. I eventually fell asleep. The following morning sharp pains woke me up. I checked my blood pressure again, it was still sky-high. But as there were no signs that labour was occurring, I decided to take the day off from work. All I needed was to rest, I told myself. On the third day I got up to the same conditions and told myself I should probably visit the hospital. I contacted a friend who works there, Lisa. I first met Lisa as a client of my cake business. One order was all it took, we became friends instantly and it felt as though I knew her forever. Lisa was the most genuine person I had ever met. Our constant conversations made her feel more like family. When I updated her on my current situation, she promptly called the labor department to have me checked by a doctor. Despite doing so, I still lingered around at home for a few additional hours. But Lisa kept calling every hour demanding I hurry over to the hospital.

I'm not sure what was really going on in my head. I just wanted to lie in bed and do nothing. Peace did not come. Instead a phone call from one of my sisters, Crystal, jolted me back into reality. Crystal and I are identical twin sisters. I suppose she thought if no one else could move me, she could. She kept asking me why I was still at home. I could hear her workmates in the background encouraging me to get to the hospital as I was in a life and death situation. Taking everyone's advice I decided to get up and get ready. As I was putting on my shoes, Crystal arrived at the house. She was smiling and that had somewhat of a calming effect on my nerves. I took up my suitcase as a mere precaution (I had no intention of this being more than a quick doctor's visit) and we headed to the hospital. When we arrived, I left my suitcase in the car and told Crystal I would call her if I needed her. In the mean time she could go pick up our children from school and then return for me.

As soon as I walked into the emergency room, the movie began to happen. It was like I was the main actress of the film... I had the strange feeling that every staff member had been anticipating my arrival. A male nurse swiftly came to my aid, asking me how far along I was in the pregnancy and what the symptoms I was experiencing were. I showed him my blood pressure home device reading and before I could say anything else, a medical orderly rushed towards me with a wheelchair. I did not have time to catch my breath before I was taken way in that same wheelchair to the labor ward. Upon my arrival to the ward, I noticed that there were five women ahead of me waiting to be assessed by a doctor. My friend Lisa appeared with the head midwife and told her of my blood pressure readings. The midwife signaled frantically to her colleagues that I was a red alert. I was put directly onto a nearby bed. A machine was strapped on me to monitor my heart rate and that of the baby, my blood pressure and the contractions. To their dismay, the blood pressure reading was even higher than my home reading. One of the nurses turned to me, her face etched with concern, she asked me, *"You want to be a dead woman? Why did you take so long to get here?"* As I pondered the answer to that question, my body became numb. My legs stiffened and started to swell rapidly. They turned purple. I was about to have a stroke.

Dr. Corbin, the assistant doctor to my Obstetrician/ Gynecologist, rushed to my bedside. Dr. Corbin did not smile much, but she had a bright countenance and she made me feel comfortable. She was accompanied by four other doctors. By this time I was going in and out of consciousness. *"Christine, listen to me, you are having a severe case of preeclampsia. We will have to take this baby immediately or both of you could die!"* was what I heard someone say. Lisa was still by my side, holding my hand. I felt like I was sinking into a dark abyss of loneliness. Her presence reassured me. She telephoned my friends and family and in no time my sisters Victoria and Crystal, as well as close friends from my church, Keisha, Leandra and Jamal, all rushed to the hospital, staying until the wee hours of the morning. They were not only anticipating the arrival of a new baby but also that I would pull through successfully. My mother, a woman with tremendous faith and a prayer warrior was constantly on the phone with my sisters to get updates on my condition. I am sure she was bombarding heaven on the behalf of me and my child. Well-wishes started flooding my phone. It occurred to me in that moment that I was never alone, and I was not alone then, in a time when I most needed others. I knew I had a family, a family that loved me dearly. And I had friends who were rooting for my success. That fresh knowledge kindled a new hope and give me a reason to push ahead.

By this time, the medical staff had put me in a small, private room to avoid any light or noise interference that would trigger my pressure. Beside the bed was a heart monitor machine, a blood pressure machine and IV stands. I was induced. During, the first process of inducement I remembered my entire body feeling as though I was on fire. I cried, asking the nurses what was causing the pain, and if they could make it stop. My cervix was still closed so I was given a balloon catheter to ripen it and I was kept under close observation.

By evening, another nurse friend by the name of Valerie came to examine me. The pains had worsened and the contractions were closer together. As Valerie gave me a pain reliever injection she said to me, *"Christine, you are a walking dead... you are lucky to still be alive"*. I felt scared and grateful at the same time. My heart melted. I was now coming into a fuller understanding of how risky my situation was. I could not believe I ignored my body and could lose my life and my baby.

My eyes would not remain open. I could scarcely make out what appeared to be the silhouettes of my sisters, Crystal and Victoria and my dear friend Lisa, all standing in the room. I smiled and then cried as pain crept up on me and my stomach began to ache again. I was feeling light headed. The pain was shooting up my back and along both sides of my body. I dosed off once more. I slept through most of the labor and didn't realize that ten hours had already passed. Victoria told me they were not allowing me to push due to a still elevated blood pressure but that if the baby did not come within two hours it would be taken through C-section surgery.

I dosed off again and I was awoken with a cramp I could not ease, a burn I could never forget. I screamed at the top of my lungs. It was time. The baby was pushing itself out and I could not stop it. I shouted for Crystal, *"Get the nurse, get the nurse NOW!"* In no time nurses came scrambling to my aid shouting *"don't push, don't push."* I responded *"it's pushing on its own, hurry up, hurry up!"*

Before their gloves were on the baby's head pop out. By the time they looked around, they only had time to lunge forward to catch the baby. The umbilical cord was dangerously wrapped around its neck. The nurses untangled the baby. Another contraction came and I scream once more. The movie of the birth of my second child was over. She was a beauty to behold. I loved her instantly.

***

It's reassuring to know that when my life and the life of my child hung in the balance, we had the support of a stadium full of supporters, cheering us on to keep pushing. It was not the most ideal of races. Some of them made it known that they did not approve of it either. But that did not stop them from seeing me through every hurdle, even when those hurdles became difficult to overcome. They kept pushing me and made me tap into strength I did not even know was inside of me.

Those are the sort of people you want to keep around you; those that have seen you in your mess and still decided to stick around; those who are willing to sacrifice a quiet evening or a favorite pass time to sit with you and help you sort through your drama. No man is an island. We all need cheerleaders, counsellors and companions to help us push forward towards our destiny. What it will require from you is a willingness to be open about hurtful experiences and to be real with others about what you are feeling. So many people give up because they think they have no one to lean on. So many commit suicide because they think others will be better off without them, or even that others would not miss them. Know this, there are people out there who have your back. My prayer is that if you don't yet see them, that God would open your eyes.

I wanted to end the pregnancy in the beginning. I thought everything was gone and I had no one who cared or loved me but I was focused on what I lost instead of what I always had. I always had supporters. I always had family and friends. I just needed to be reminded of that, and because of that, the birth of my child was not only her own birth but the birth of a new me, a birth of new beginnings. Out of any mess, depression and feelings of loneliness can come new life and a new you when you find the right someone to lean on.

Chapter Seven

Uprooting Bitterness

Moving on is not always easy. The birth of my child signified a new chapter in my life had begun... but the work of picking up a pen and writing still fell to me. There were things I needed to work at, foremost among them, bitterness. Writer and bible teacher Erin Davis in one of her "Revive our Hearts" blogs[6], described bitterness this way. *"Bitterness isn't one of those big, flashy sins that you can see growing above the surface of our hearts. It may not show off like anger or produce big ol' hunks of rotten fruit like disobedience.*

Bitterness is a sleeper sin. It grows beneath the surface, down deep in the soil of our hearts".

Have you ever unexpectedly bitten into a bitter fruit? Your face almost immediately begins to twist, it feels like if your throat shuts off and you just want to hurl the contents from your mouth. Even after you have done so, you may still find yourself spitting and trying to wipe away the remains of the aftertaste. That is how awful bitterness is, and that should be our response to getting it out of our lives.

Bitterness is resentment boiled over and left to ferment. You may no longer be angry at a person, in fact you may be able to smile when you see them. But if that person's name comes up in a conversation, you can't help but remind others what that person did to you. In fact, you often replay in your mind the hurt they caused you. You blame them for the breakdown of the relationship. You blame them for misery that has befallen you. The person could be long dead, but you are still blaming them for what is happening to you. Today many persons are in hospital beds, not because of poor eating or lack of exercise, but because of bitterness which can manifest itself physically in the form of sicknesses such as strokes, ulcers, even cancer. Have you ever been around someone who always has something bad to say about someone else? And they try to get you to join them in slandering that person? Their speaking reflects the type of hearts they have, hearts overrun with roots of bitterness.

All of us have been hurt by the actions or words of another. Perhaps your mother criticized you repeatedly when you were a child, a colleague sabotaged a work project which cost you to lose lots of money, or even lose your job unfairly. Perhaps your spouse had an affair, or the love of your life went away and left you with promises of the family he intended to build with you… but the months you were waiting turned into years. Now he has his own family and never once looked back to say sorry.

Years may pass us by, but these wounds can leave us with lasting feelings of deep-seated hurt, anger and feelings of betrayal. How then can we stop these feelings from finding a home in our hearts, from being swallowed up by bitterness and sense of injustice at the hands of others? We must alter our attitude to free ourselves of this bondage, we must develop a new way of looking at our past, present and future and most importantly, we must learn to forgive those that hurt us in order to let go of our retaliatory rage so that we can move on.

***

My child was resembling her absent father more and more each day... and though I love her with all my heart, seeing his face in her hurt liked hell because I hated him, but more so because I still loved him. It wasn't the type of love that caused my heart to throb and my knees to get weak. I knew better by now. But it was the type of love where memories lingered, where scenes of what was and what may have been replayed in my mind. It was the type of love that was like a raw sore, a love that pained me.

The immediate aftermath of our storm of a relationship was just as devastating as the storm itself. One day as I was sitting in my TV room my phone rang. It was a voice I had never heard asking me how I was doing and how the baby was growing (my daughter had not yet arrived). I was hesitant to answer the stranger's questions until he introduced himself as Paul's friend. Paul had travelled a week or two prior to this phone call and he had asked his friend to check on me. Although I was angry at Paul for not being man enough to let me know he was traveling I figured he cared because of this. His friend went on to explain how Paul was going through a hard time and I needed to take it easy as he had a lot going on but would make good on his promises to provide some baby furniture. *He has a lot going on? What about me? Are you seriously telling me this?* I smiled sarcastically and hung up the telephone.

Well into my third trimester of pregnancy Paul started to request a DNA test to prove that he was indeed the father of our child. By this time talk was spreading and people were trying to convince him that Mark was the father. I guess he tried to hold out for as long as he could but the chatter finally got to him and he backed away completely. But it wasn't just that. One day a "friend" approached me to question me about Mark. He said that Mark was the cause of the situation between Paul and me and that I should give Paul the DNA test he requested as I would need help with the child. *"Help? If he hasn't helped me for seven months what makes you or him think that I will need help now?"* I yelled at him. I could only take so much, the resentment in me was brewing over. I was angry as hell. Horns were growing out of my head by the time Paul's son decided to "check in on me". The formalities out of the way, he began asking me about the baby and then about the whereabouts of the baby's daddy. I gritted my teeth and responded, *"my dear, my baby daddy is your daddy."* By this time I knew there was some talk he had gotten wind of. *"Are you sure it is my dad's one? Aren't you getting married or something along that line?"* he facetiously asked. I left him with a piece of my mind and hung up the phone.

When it wasn't from Paul's side, I had persons seemingly bringing me well wishes but their real motives were to defend Mark. I was accused of treating Mark badly and rejecting his efforts to make a relationship between us work. I don't deny this entirely because it is partly and sadly true. But what made me recoil was when I heard how he promised to take care of the baby as if it were his own. *Really? Then why would you suggest I get an abortion?* I heard about how I forced him into giving me a ring. *I forced??? That piece of... no wonder my blood pressure was soaring through the roof!*

By the time our daughter was born, Paul had taken to telling everyone who would listen that the child was not his own and he would not be supporting her. He could not simply move on. He had to drag my name and character in the mud to make him feel better about himself I suppose. I was mad. I was so mad that I had thoughts of doing something to hurt him. Something I know I would regret. It was trying for me. Bringing home a newborn baby is a hard enough job already, without having to deal with emotional dead weight. I longed for my heart to be healed but it was like a big gaping wound. With the encouragement of family and friends, I began to pray every night for Paul, asking God to soften his heart. To be honest I did this less for him and more for me, as a way to help me forgive him and move on. I also hoped that my daughter would have a relationship with her father.

Praying for him and working through on my own with our daughter might have been all I would have done in the first few months of her life, had it not been for the continuing stream of calls from people questioning me about the identity of the baby's true father. Already not all there emotionally, this talk was like an exposed wire that kept tripping in my head. I felt that if I did not take some sort of action, I would lose my mind. I decided to lay out my case before my lawyer. I was going to put Paul in court. It was not about the money. You may say I was being spiteful. Maybe a part of me was. But for me, it was mostly a matter of calling him out for being a coward. Instead of blaming me and blackening my name in the minds of his friends and family, he would have to face the fact that his decision not to be involved in his child's life fell squarely at his feet.

Weeks after, Paul and I were summoned to

Court. He was hopping mad when he found out. I admit I got some satisfaction from his reaction. The morning of the hearing, I arrived at the court early. The court yard was filled with many people, some laughing, others fretting about the other party involved. As I look around once more, what I noticed was the lack of support from men when it came to raising their children. *Why did it need to reach this stage? Why did one have to put a man in court to pay attention to the child he helped conceive?* Our names were called. As I entered the court room the atmosphere was tense. My lawyer sat on the left. Paul had chosen to represent himself. We both stood in the middle of the courtroom as the presiding judge sat on her platform. Just below her was the secretary. As she proceeded, she stated the nature of the case and asked Paul to pronounce his daughter's name. He did not. The judge then asked him if the child was his. Paul did not even flinch in his response, *"I don't know Ma'am, that is what I would like to know."* The judge ordered that an appointment be made for a DNA test to be taken.

Court was adjourned. In less than three weeks the results of that test were back and our second appearance in court took place. We stood once more before the same judge and Paul was asked to read the results of the DNA test out loud. *"Who is the father of this child?"* the judge asked once more. I stared at Paul from half way across the room, I stared at him so intensely he must have felt holes burning at the side of his face. Paul answered *"I am the father"* and had the audacity to appear shocked.

The weeks to follow were in no way impacted by this new "revelation". Paul still made no attempt to see his daughter nor did he help me financially with her expenses. I keep hoping that one day that will change, not for me but for our daughter's sake. Still, I cannot allow his absence to hold me or our child emotionally hostage.

***

Overcoming hurt caused by broken relationship requires time and divine intervention. Our own effort is certainly required in the healing process. We must want to be healed. We must want to walk in freedom. Help cannot come to someone who is hell-bent on nursing pain. Not even God will wrestle misery out of the hands of someone who chooses to cuddle it with great affection. So how do we go about uprooting bitterness from our lives? As I said, we have a part to play and God has a part to play.

Our part in uprooting bitterness is to first acknowledge that it is there and secondly, to be willing to part with it. The same David that declares in our well-loved Psalms 139:11 that we are *fearfully and wonderfully* made by God, says to that same God in verse 23-24 *"Search me, O God, and know my heart; Try me and know my anxious thoughts; And see if there be any hurtful way in me, And lead me in the everlasting way.*[7] God sees the very depths of our heart and if we ask Him to, He is will show us what is inside. Sometimes He shows us even when we do not ask, or he may use other people to tell us. Some of us, instead of acknowledging the bitterness in our hearts, deny that it exists, and continue on a path of laying the blame at everyone else's feet except ours. But for those who are willing to part with those things in our heart which are offensive to God, the *Searcher and Mender of hearts* promises to help us through the process.

So what is God's part? He cuts away the bad in us, and prunes what remains so that we can be better versions of ourselves. There is another biblical story about a Gardener and his vineyard. In John 15, Jesus describes himself as a vine and his Father as the gardener. We who walk in relationship with God are branches on that vine. He goes on to say, "*Every branch in me that beareth not fruit he taketh away: and every branch that beareth fruit, he purgeth it, that it may bring forth more fruit"*. Any gardener knows that in order to get the best out of your plants, you will be required from time to time to cut off dead branches or withering leaves. Sometimes you cut even the branches that may look healthy, but in doing so, you allow the plant to better thrive so that it bears even more leaves, fruits and blossoms. Alternatively, think about that time you went to the hairdresser and she said to you, "your hair is unhealthy, you need to cut off all these dead ends". You may be sad, especially if your hair has considerable length. But notice what happens when she cuts the hair. Almost immediately you begin to see changes. The hair begins to breathe. There is a bounce to it and it appears to have more volume. In the days and weeks to come, the growth of that hair is more than what you may have experienced in the months passed.

So it is with us when we allow God to completely uproot harmful bitterness from our lives. It may pain us to go through the process of letting go of what we have grown attached to, but the end result is that our souls can breathe once more, the air around is no longer toxic and we are free to grow and thrive in the best God has for us.

Chapter Eight

Guarding Our Hearts

The lessons I learned and which were outlined in the previous chapters, if applied wholly in your life, will ensure that you guard your heart. Why does your heart need to be guarded? Proverbs 4:23 tells us to, "*Above all else, guard your heart, for everything you do flows from it*"[8]. Your heart is the central command of your life. It determines the course of your life, the decisions you take and consequently, the results of those decisions that will either propel you to fulfil your purpose or delay you, sidetrack you, even imprison you. We can look around today and see the consequences of hearts which have been hijacked by the enemy called anger, or lust, or pride. We see the results of unguarded hearts that fell to the sword of bitterness, selfishness, envy and greed. People are driven to hurt and murder. Homes are destroyed because of abuse and adultery. People see prostitution and drug pushing as honorable jobs. Entire nations are at war with each other because of the pride, envy and greed of a few.

As women, we will spare ourselves from so much pain if we are careful in the way we handle our hearts. Debra Fileta, a professional counselor in dating, marriage and relationship issues, stated that *guarding your hearts mean protecting the deepest parts of who you are from anyone who can cause it harm.*[9] Accept the fact that everyone who comes smiling and bearing gifts does not mean you well. Others may mean you well but are not emotionally mature enough to be entrusted with your heart.

Sooner or later, they will drop it, break it and destroy it in frustration. There is no such thing as a "casual" relationship when the heart is involved. Everything concerning the heart is a serious matter. Sometimes we wait until we are fully submerged in the waters of a love affair to try to assess the matters of our heart. This is not wise. Even as the first sign of danger is signaled by the watchman on the guard wall because he has a wider view and is able to pick up threats from afar, the task of guarding our heart should be happening way before someone approaches us and knocks on our heart's gates. You can be real, you can be genuine and honest, but never without the anchor of boundaries and the weight of wisdom, let your guard down. Ladies, avoid making someone the center of your life. It's time to begin guarding your heart.

***

Except the LORD build the house, they labour in vain that build it: except the LORD keep the city, the watchman waketh but in vain.[10] Stabbing pains in my chest awoke me a few days after. I could not move from my bed. Tears flooded my eyes and soon soaked my pillow. I asked myself. *"Why me? Did he not love me? Will my daughter ever know her father? How can I move on? Am I going to die of this broken heart?"* A feeling of grief overwhelmed me and in that moment I started to question God, *"Oh God, if you loved me, how can you let this happen to me?"* My body felt so weak and I burst out in tears all over again. How much can a heart handle? I definitely was broken. All my prayers, all my hopes, all my dreams, flushed quickly down the toilet. I had believed that taking Paul to court would have solved the issue. But it did not. It did not solve the issue because the real issue was not the fact that he dropped my heart and broke it into a million pieces. The real issue was that I gave it to him in the first place... that I was so reckless with my heart. I had built on a poor foundation. How could I build on a poor foundation and expect the house of my life to stand when tested. I broke down in tears again. I now saw that my only hope was to turn back to God and ask Him to heal my heart once more. I prayed a simple prayer, *"God, I need you now more than ever, I need your help through this difficult time."* I cried loudly once again and felt I would choke to death on my grief.

And then something interrupted my hysterical wailing. It was the crying sound of my baby who lay next to me. I managed to compose myself and as I unwrapped my sheet from over my head, a peace came over me. There she was, now she looked up at me with a smile. I returned her smile, a little embarrassed that I was proving to be a bigger baby than her that morning. And then I sensed God speaking to me. *After the storm, there comes a smile. Weeping may endure for a night but joy comes in the morning.* The storm was over. The night was through. I needed to let go of the past and focus on what was before me. I needed to forgive myself. I needed to stop blaming him or myself. As

I sat on my bed acknowledging these things, I took up my Bible and opened it. The first thing my eyes landed one was this: *"The LORD is close to the brokenhearted and saves those who are crushed in spirit."* Psalms 34:18. I cried once again, this time it was not tears of pain but tears of joy to know that God was still there for me.

In the weeks and months to follow, I became surer of the fact that everything happens for a reason and the separation was very much necessary. God in his mercy, had saved me from a storm that could have killed me. God give me back hope. But I also had to learn from this experience. I had to refortify the walls of my heart. I knew I was still vulnerable and I knew that in this vulnerable state, I was likely to make unwise decisions. What steps could I take to avoid going down this path again? I had to look back once more… this time, not with regret, but with the guidance of God to show me the breaches in the walls of my heart. I pulled out my journal and began to write.

***

We must prepare ourselves for a relationship long before a man comes into our lives, if not, we may find that our emotions force us into less than ideal situations. You must define what is less than ideal for you. For me, less than ideal is placing myself in a situation where I walk in conflict with the core values on which I wish to base by own life. One such core value is family life as God ordains it. I refuse to lay down my value and my virtue again for someone whose version of family life is "shacking up", having multiple sexual partners and refusing to commit wholeheartedly to the sanctity of marriage. I refuse give away myself to someone who is not willing to pay the price for me (*they want to have the goods but don't want to put a ring on my finger*). I refuse to listen to anyone who tells me that God's standards for me are a waste of time. I refuse to share my life romantically with anyone who does not see himself as accountable to God for my life.

Ladies, you must determine for yourselves what you will refuse to let enter into your heart. You must determine that in these areas, *I will guard my heart and will only consent to letting down my guard when I am convinced that that person is no threat.* Write down your standards. Be very clear in your mind what they are at all times and do not hesitate to communicate them to anyone who approaches. Ensure they are in alignment with the standards God has for you. God's opinion matters most because it is truth and because it is the best on offer to ensure you carry out your unique purpose.

My experiences have brought me to this conclusion: A woman that pays attention to God's subtle warnings, commits to walking in sexually purity because she honors her body as God's temple, refuses to tie herself emotionally to dead weight but instead anchors her emotions on the solid rock of God's Word, a woman that submits herself to wise counsel and does not make room in her heart for bitterness which will poison her and those who come close to her, such a woman stands the greatest chance of guarding her heart and maintaining her freedom.

I encourage you ladies to use wisdom and be cautious in handling your heart. Be strong enough to love but smart enough to guard your heart and wise enough to know who you let in. Not everyone is deserving of it. Every mistake you have made, every moment of weakness you have felt, every terrible thing that has ever happened to you, GROW from it. Your past experiences do not determine who you are or where you go from here, your past experiences prepare you for who you are yet to become.....a beautiful, powerful, woman of worth.

Inspirational Quotes & Daily Affirmations

Anger, Resentment and Jealousy doesn't change the heart of others it only changes yours. *Shannon Alder*

I now choose to release all hurt and resentment. *Louise Hay*

Know your worth. Know the difference between what you're getting and what you deserve.

I am worth being loved, I am worth being

cherished, I am worth an effort. I am worth being someone's everything.

If you find yourself constantly trying to prove your worth to someone you have already forgotten your value

I am not an option. I am a priority

I am worth more than I think.

Don't rely on someone else for your happiness and self-worth. Only you can be responsible for that. If you can't love and respect yourself – no one else will be able to make that happen. Accept who you are – completely; the good and the bad – and make changes as YOU see fit – not because you think someone else wants you to be different. – *Stacey Charter*

It is not what you think you are that's holding you back, it's what you think you are not.

Self respect, self worth and self love all start with Self. Stop looking outside of yourself for your value. – *Rob Liano*

I am worth it, always was and always will be

To be beautiful means to be yourself. You don't need to be accepted by others. You need to accept yourself!

You survived what you thought would break you. Now straighten that crown and move forward like the queen you are.

References

1. Quote taking from Ebrahim Aseem. Website

2. New International Version (NIV)

3. Quote from tele-evangelist Joyce Meyers.Website https://www.joycemeyer.org/articles/ea.aspx?article =we_cant_rely_on_emotions (This article is taken from Joyce's four-CD series, *Why Do I Feel the Way I Feel?.*)

4. Excerpt from **Marmion**, an epic poem by Walter Scott, published 1808.

5. New Living Translation (NLT)

6. Quote from writer and bible teacher Erin Davis. Website https://www.reviveourhearts.com/true-woman/blog/four-ways-to-spot-a-bitter-root/

(Posted Sept 15, 2014)

7. New American Standard (NAS)

8. New International Version (NIV)

9. Quote from Debra Fileta. Website

10. Psalms 127:1 King James Version (KJV)

Appreciation

I wish to extend my sincerest gratitude to First God the Father, the Son and the Holy Spirit who directed me in writing this book. I also extend my thanks to my mom Diana Nicholls, my Sisters Victoria and Crystal Nicholls who encouraged me and stood by me during my difficult times.

I am also grateful for my friends Keisha Rodgers, Tonya Stephens, Selena King, Debrol Greaves and Secorah Small who constantly supported me during the process of this book.

To my Graphic Artist Shanice Bourne-Jordan and my Editor RuthMoisa Alleyne who made this possible and worked endlessly with me, I do thank you.

I also extend a special thank you to my daughters

Janiyah & J'Leiah Nicholls who were my inspiration in writing this book.

About the Author

Miss Christine Nicholls currently resides in Barbados and was born to Barbadian parents Diana & Guy Nicholls. She is a single mother of two daughters Janiyah and J'Leiah Nicholls. Her experiences have allowed her to be an advocate for all women as she firmly believes that one's past and one's present circumstances do not have to determine one's destiny. A self-starter and industrious young lady, Christine turned a love for baking into a thriving home-business now operating under the name, House Of Cakes.

www.ingramcontent.com/pod-product-compliance
Lightning Source LLC
Chambersburg PA
CBHW070520030426
42337CB00016B/2034